Soft Landing
Lessons I learned about life, through death

By Gabrielle Elise Jimenez

Death is sad, it can be painful, and it is hard but it doesn't have to be dark, or scary or ugly or done alone. Prior to becoming a hospice nurse I saw a lot of death, but I never felt death, I never understood death, I never let it crawl up inside me to the point that I totally and completely got it. I have done that now, I embrace it like a warm comforting hug and my goal is to help families and loved ones to have a less painful experience. With life comes death, sometimes after a long full life, sometimes not. But it is always emotional, personal, intimate and private and should be treated as such.

Acknowledgment

I dedicate this book to all of the friends and family members of the patients I have helped provide a soft landing for. I thank you for trusting them in my care. I thank you for sharing them with me. I thank you for opening your hearts to me and allowing me into your private moments. I cherish them and all of you more than you will ever know and I am a better nurse because of each and every one of you.

To my kids, I want you to know that bringing you into this world was the most amazing thing I have ever done. I am so very thankful and grateful you are in my life. I am proud of you, I respect you and I love you with every ounce of my being. If I can teach you anything, it is to embrace your life and every single moment and to love fully and completely.

I also want to give a very special thank you to Dr. Gary Pasternak. I respect you, I admire you, I strive to be more like you and I thank you for all of your guidance, trust and friendship.
I love you!

Whenever I tell someone I am a Hospice Nurse, I always get THAT look, which is followed by; "it must be so hard to work around death all the time". It is hard; it is the toughest job I have ever done. But while I do see a lot of death, what I also see is LIFE and love, family, and so many different cultures. I also see spirituality in a way that completely inspires me. I see families who have such strong faith and who pray with every ounce of their being. This inspires me.

When I first meet a family, I tell them that I can't change the outcome, I can't make their loved one better, and I can't heal them, but, I can promise them that I will make every effort to ensure they are comfortable, that their pain is relieved, that they do not suffer and that they never die alone. This is a promise I strive to keep with every single patient I have the honor of caring for. I take a hold of their hands, I look them straight in the eyes, I wrap my heart around theirs and I assure them that I will do my best to provide a soft landing.

Caring for someone at the end of life is an honor, an honor I take seriously and to heart. This is the most difficult, most intimate, most personal time of their lives and it deserves to be treated with the utmost respect and care.

I wasn't always a Hospice nurse though; in fact it never even crossed my mind. At the age of 40-something I completely changed my life. This book is about my experiences as a hospice nurse. I will share why and how I started, what inspires me, and what I have learned thus far. I will share my perspective, my heart, my soul and my passion. And I will share some of the stories of patients that continue to hold space in my heart. To respect their privacy and HIPPA laws, I have changed a few things, but the message is still there and that is what matters most to me. And in my heart... I know who they are and I always will.

For about 15 years I managed commercial real estate in Silicon Valley; one of the most expensive pieces of property in Silicon Valley to be exact. I wore the fancy clothes; the high heels and I made the big bucks. Okay not really, I mean… I made a whole lot more than I do now, but it wasn't quite the "big bucks". But I felt fancy. I felt important. I felt like I had a big job with a big title and I felt pretty badass.

Around 9/11, "safety" became a serious issue everywhere and the property I was managing needed a safety program. I had absolutely no knowledge of what this might entail but I took on the project. I created a Life Safety Plan, an Emergency Evacuation Plan, and I scheduled safety classes and fire drills regularly. I worked with the Police and Fire Departments on the best ways to keep our tenants safe in an emergency. I studied and learned all of the OSHA guidelines and regulations and became very interested in safety. I created a pretty impressive safety plan for two commercial buildings and several hundred people.

I left the property management field and went into safety. I became a Safety Coordinator first for a commercial construction company and then for a steel company. I helped raise their ExMod, I brought everyone up to code and I became pretty darn good at safety. And then I was laid off.

At this time I had a friend who was diagnosed with Prostate Cancer and was put on Hospice with less than 6 months to live. This was a man who I had always admired. He was one of the kindest, funniest, loveliest people I knew and I was lucky he chose me to be his friend. This diagnosis was something I didn't understand. I don't even think I took it as seriously as I should have. I had lost both parents and several friends to cancer over the years but I think I somehow managed to put a wall up between myself and truly reacting to or understanding death. As my mother used to say… I saw things through rose-colored glasses; always trying to see the positive side and never truly seeing things for what they actually were. Death was not something I understood or had ever really let inside. I think it would be very honest to say that I was almost in denial when it came to death.

My friend was dying and his wife was struggling and I don't think I understood what she was going through until one day, after I had been laid off, she asked if I could come help take care of him so she could work. I said yes without hesitation. I spent time with him while his illness slowly took his life. I helped bathe him, feed him, monitor him and I even slept in a bed next to his so I could respond to anything he needed. I watched as Hospice Nurses came in and gave him medications and assessed him. I watched as someone I loved was struggling with the most difficult thing a person will ever endure. Death. I watched my friend lose her husband. My heart ached for both of them. My heart ached for me.

Each day I was lucky enough to spend with him was one more day that I was absolutely certain I was meant to care for people at the end of their lives.

After he passed away and at the age of 40-something, I enrolled in a class to become a Certified Nursing Assistant (CNA). I was one of the oldest in the class. I was intimidated, and honestly a little embarrassed but I was determined to do this. My CNA teacher was amazing, she taught me so much. She was also a special needs teacher for children and allowed us to come in and do some of our clinical training with the kids. That was incredibly heart warming. I got to spend time with kids with Down Syndrome, kids who were Autistic, kids who were unable to walk or breathe or eat without machines, and kids who couldn't speak, eat, or laugh. And yet they were the strongest, bravest and most inspiring young people I had ever met. These kids reminded me to lighten up a little, to appreciate everything, to be more patient, and to be more kind. They gave me lessons that helped mold me into the nurse I am now. I considered working with kids as a nurse but I knew my heart couldn't handle it. I had to be honest with myself and knew this was not the direction I was meant to go.

After I received my Certified Nursing Assistant (CNA) certificate, I continued moving forward and I received my Acute Care certificate, and then my Home Health Aid (HHA). I started working for families caring for their loved ones. I worked at first for a company that sent me out to different homes every day. I would spend a few hours with complete strangers; usually as a companion. I spent most of my time with the elderly.

During this time, one of my daughter's friends, at the age of 23, was in a horrible accident. He ended up spending 19 days in the hospital while we all sat vigil at his bedside and in the waiting room. His death struck us all very hard. It is something we will never truly get over. He was the ultimate gentleman, the sweetest young man I had ever known. He touched us all.

It was during the time we were all sitting vigil for him that I met his family and friends. I was introduced to a family that needed a caregiver for their grandfather. I started working for this family and after a few months started taking care of their grandmother as well. I took them to doctor appointments, I bathed them, I cooked for them, I provided comfort and support and we became friends.

As I watched them start to decline, I felt like there was more I could do for them. I wanted to understand their illnesses, their medications and their treatments. I wanted to do more for them. I wanted to be a nurse.

And this… is where my life completely changed.

After researching a few nursing schools, I finally found the one that made most sense to me. I went in to the school and met with their financial aid department and found out exactly what I needed to do to enroll in nursing school. The gal I met with was the angel on my shoulder from day one and is someone I still consider a friend.

She helped me qualify for financial aid. She signed me up for the entrance exam and she sent me on my way to make nursing school happen.

I took the entrance exam.
I got the phone call that I passed.
This kinda blew my mind, I won't lie. I was shocked. The one thing I was absolutely not good at was school, so this was a big deal for me.

Passing meant I was going to be enrolled into the pre requisite classes and I would be a nursing school student. I was pretty excited. Until they said they needed my high school diploma. I had never graduated from high school. My bubble was now burst and I felt so ashamed and embarrassed and sad. The financial aid gal never gave up on me, she refused to allow me to see each thing as an obstacle, despite how big they were and how often they seemed to block my way. She encouraged me to take the GED and would save a spot for me in the class. I had two months to make this happen.

I reached out to the school where I had gotten my CNA. I reached out to my instructor and the people I got to know there. They all helped me. They took their personal time to tutor me. I took the 5 tests and I received my GED about a week before nursing school was about to start. I did it! I graduated high school and enrolled in college in the same week.

The family I was working for kept me on while I went to school. They were flexible with my hours, they allowed me to study and do homework and they encouraged and supported me every single step of the way. It was during this time that one of them passed. It was my first time with death while on this path. My heart felt differently. I had cared for him for over a year so I was clearly attached but it was more than that. It was at this time where death made sense to me, that it became a part of the process, that it was inevitable but it absolutely did not need to be dark, or scary or lonely. His death was peaceful. His death was painless. He did not die alone.

I remember receiving the phone call. I dropped everything and went straight to their home. I walked in to see their entire family gathered together in their living room; surrounding the Matriarch, "Grandma", my friend, who just lost her husband of 60+ years. Their love was a crazy love; sometimes chaotic, but always a loving, devoted and loyal love. She was in good hands.

I walked into the other room, where he lay in his hospital bed. I dropped down to my knees next to the bed, I grabbed a hold of his chubby wonderful hands and I said, "Hi Luis, it's me "Lee Lee" (which was his nickname for me) and I cried. And I cry as I write this too, because I gave my heart to him, I cared for him and I loved him. I had to say goodbye to him and that was hard. This was my first patient that I provided care for until he passed away. I knew this was going to be the hard part for me in the career I was choosing.

After he passed away it was just his wife and I and we spent a lot of time talking about her husband, their life together and working through her grief. This was my first real lesson on being fully present at a death. I learned how to be fully present for someone else. I learned how to listen with my heart. I learned the difference between offering words and offering an ear. I learned that not everything is about me.

Starting nursing school meant making some changes, big changes. I had to move out of my little house I had rented for so many years. I sold, gave and threw away just about everything I had hoarded over the years. This was tough. My house was my safe place, my friend's safe place, the place my son and daughter and their friends grew up... so many memories. The stuff I saved was placed in storage and I rented a room from a friend at an incredibly generously low rate. They let me bring my cat and my other wonderful friends took in my dog. This was the only way I could make this happen. I had to give up a lot to reduce my expenses and responsibilities in order to truly focus on this journey. And I was broke. I was only working part time and paying for nursing school. My whole life changed. But boy did my friends rally. I honestly could not have done this if it were not for my friends. They supported me emotionally and in many ways financially. Some loaned me money to get by, and a group of them threw a fundraiser for me at a local bar we all hung out at. Theirs was a generous, kind and wonderful love and I will be forever grateful for it. I was studying so much, I was no longer able to hang out like before and while I think it frustrated them, they were patient with me and took whatever time I was able to give. Which was not very much.

Nursing school was not easy. There were so many obstacles. My angel in the Financial Aid department continued to support and encourage me, my family and friends encouraged me, and when my friends whom I was renting from made the decision to sell their house and I needed a place to live (again), my boyfriend at the time offered me to move in, rent free and took care of me all through nursing school. He gave me a place to study, he cooked meals for me, he held my hand and hugged me when I didn't think I could do this. We did not end up staying together, but I will be forever grateful for the role he played in helping me get through nursing school. I know it was because of all of them that I managed to get past the obstacles with very few scratches.

It was also during this time that I discovered I was dyslexic; it sure would have been nice if I had discovered this earlier... like in high school!!! Anyway, this made studying and test taking really tough. I received some support from other friends who had been through this and got some great test taking tips, which helped a lot. The school also helped me by allowing me a quiet space to take tests.

There was a lot of drama in nursing school, mostly because of the age of the other students. Initially it was fine but quickly into the program the gossip, the bully behavior and the meanness became very obvious, it was so distracting for me. I had a very small few that I considered "friends". This was the loneliest part of the journey. There were many days that I felt really alone on campus, some days I didn't want to go back. But I did, every single day. I remember sitting alone on breaks, as most of the other students ate together, chatted together and studied together. It was a struggle for me to walk into the classroom every day and be ignored. I vowed I would never treat anyone this way or allow anyone to be treated this way. Every single day I made an effort to get in their good graces, when what I really wanted to do was to give them a spanking and a time out! But I did it for myself and for our group. We finally got to a place where this behavior became a distant memory and Nursing school resumed.

My next big obstacle was when I failed the Psyche midterm. They gave me another chance to take it but I failed it again. This meant I could not finish with my class. This was heartbreaking. That day, when I found out I did not pass was the same day they called me back in the office and told me I could not complete the course with my class and would have to come back and redo the last module of the course. I was devastated. I wanted to quit. I felt so incredibly defeated. But I agreed to come back when the next session started. I still went to their graduation. It took everything I had to sit in the audience and watch the group of students I had been with for so many months graduate from a program I worked so hard for. I congratulated them. I hugged them. I even took pictures with some of them. And I cried all the way home because I was not one of them. I had called my boyfriend from the parking lot of the school, I was in tears, he said "baby come home". When I walked in the door, he just held me and let me cry. I cried a lot. He told me "you will pass it the next time".

Each time I explained to someone that I had to go back and take over the last module, the pain in my gut increased. I was so embarrassed. Every time I said it with a smile and always tried to have a really good attitude about it, but the truth is, it was probably one of my hardest personal losses to work though and overcome. I faked it each time someone asked me about it.

For three months I studied everything I could get my hands on. I practiced studying using tips I learned online for people with Dyslexia. I took online practice tests over and over until I almost memorized the answers. I was ready to go back to nursing school and I was determined to go full speed ahead and kick this last module in the butt.

I was still providing care for the woman I started out with as a CNA. We spent a lot of time together. We were very close. She never gave up on me and wouldn't let me give up on myself. I made flash cards and she quizzed me. She would say to me "don't worry about me right now, you need to study" and I would. And then school started back up and I started the last module over again.

The new class of students welcomed me in, they invited me to join their study groups and they included me completely. They were wonderful. I helped tutor some of them and encouraged and motivated those who were nervous or scared. We were a team. We took our final test and we all passed. We passed nursing school. Together!!! Graduating nursing school was probably the proudest moment I have ever experienced (besides being a mommy). I put on that graduation cap and gown and I sat on the stage with my classmates as I looked out into the audience. I couldn't see them because of the lights, but I knew that my kids, my family, and all of my friends were out there feeling just as proud of me as I was feeling for myself. When I walked across that stage and accepted my diploma, I felt bigger than life. At almost 50 years young I was a graduate of nursing school. With honors!!!

I signed up to take my NCLEX as soon as I was able to and I studied every single day. I remember walking into the testing room; I was a sweaty, terrified mess. I scooted my chair into a little booth, I put my headphones on and I pushed "start". There were questions I had no idea what the heck they were talking about, things I never studied, calculations that didn't make sense and question, after question that left me feeling absolutely confident I failed. I walked out of the testing place feeling defeated.

There were tricks people talked about to find out early if you passed or not and yes, I tried them, but I had also read that those were false so I had to accept that all I could do was wait. And I waited for a little over a month; every day checking my mail.

I remember the day I went to get my mail. I grabbed the stack of envelopes, sifting through them, hoping that maybe today would be the day. And there it was; the letter from the Nursing Licensing Board. I was so scared to open it. For my entire life I believed I was destined to fail, that I was not worthy of anything good. No one should ever feel this way and unfortunately I spent most of my life with this mindset. As I stood there staring at the envelope, I went back to the past few years that led me here, how hard I worked, how well I've done despite the odds and I knew that whatever was in that envelope would NOT deter me from achieving greatness. I would not give up on myself. So I opened it and there were at least 1000 words but all I saw, was "congratulations you passed the NCLEX exam" and I cried. And I smiled. And I laughed. And I cried some more. I did it. I actually really did it. I couldn't wait to shout it from the tops of every mountain. I was so proud of myself.

I ran into the house and told my boyfriend. I think he was as happy as I was. He had such pride in his eyes. That feeling of knowing that someone is proud of you, is something you hold onto forever. This might sound really silly, but that day he posted on his FB "I am so proud of my girlfriend, she passed her NCLEX exam and is now a licensed nurse" (or something like that). I will never forget that day, that gesture or the way it made me feel.

Unfortunately my life had been a pattern of really high high's that always followed by a low, low. This time was no different. I did pass the exam and I qualified to receive my nursing license, however, 10 years prior I decided to drink and drive and got a DUI. It was ten years before this and I hadn't gotten even a parking ticket since but that didn't matter. No one wants to give someone with a DUI a license to pass out medications. So for several months I fought the State, I begged, I wrote letters, my friends wrote letters. I was sure, once again, that this was just not going to happen.

But then it did. They decided that this should not get in my way of becoming a nurse and they promised to send my license within the next 3-4 weeks.

And I became a nurse. The feeling of holding my license in my hand is like nothing I had ever experienced. Pride. Relief. Honor. My life was truly about to change.

Applying for jobs felt a little surreal. I had gone through the process, I passed the test, I had the license, but actually applying for a job as a nurse was kind of bizarre. I really didn't have any actual experience as a licensed nurse. I had a kind and compassionate heart. I cared for people all of my life. I was hired to care for people. Yep. I was a nurse. Now I just had to convince the person on the other side of the desk.

I applied at skilled nursing and assisted living facilities, hospitals and home care providers. There were many positions available. I was offered two jobs at the same time. One was at a Board and Care facility, which just didn't fit what I was hoping for. The other was a skilled nursing facility, with 45 patients and the perfect opportunity for me to learn how to be a nurse. It was a fast paced job, which I was intimated by and a little bit scared of, but I accepted the job and was ready to take it all on.

I had to do three weeks of training, so the family I was working for adjusted my schedule to make it work. It was a lot to learn and everything had rules and regulations I had to abide by. So many things I didn't know. I had to document and initial and sign for every single thing, which proved to be frustrating and overwhelming but I did it. And at the end of the three weeks, I was ready to go on the floor on my own. I was really happy about this.

But, with a heavy heart I had to leave the lady I cared for. They knew this time was coming and although they were sad, they knew I needed to go out and be a nurse. This family was so supportive of my journey, and was very instrumental in my getting this far. We cried on my last day, it was hard for me to leave her. *I went and visited her frequently though after that… until she passed away a year later.*

I started working as a nurse. I was on the floor, with 15 patients of my own, and unfortunately the other nurses were not very helpful and made things very difficult for me to find my way. I persevered. The team of CNA's and HHA's were always very helpful and supportive though and helped to fill in the blanks when I had that "lost and confused" look on my face. I worked a lot of hours and all the worst shifts but it was all worth it because I was a nurse.

I struggled with the way their resident's were treated. They were basically ignored, dismissed and left alone often. There was one Hospice patient on the floor I worked that lay in his bed day after day with no one sitting with him or visiting with him. I would spend my breaks in his room. I would talk with him, read to him, and attend to his needs. And I was scolded for it. I didn't understand this. There was no explanation. I was simply told by my supervisor that my breaks were not to be spent with the residents/patients. I asked if I could spend more time with him when I was on the floor but was told that medication pass was my priority and if I had time I could check in on him. But medication pass was my whole job. The minute I finally passed all the meds, I would have to start back to the first resident/patient again and pass the next round. There was one resident that for whatever reason, the staff was not fond of and actually avoided her. I would see her call light lit and ask why no one had gone in there. They told me to check on her. (she wasn't on my floor) She was an older lady; a little needy I guess you could say, mostly just lonely. She was very specific in her needs and had a condescending way with her words. I was not offended, nor was I put off. In fact I welcomed the challenge and although it was always a struggle to leave, I responded to her needs and listened to her. Of course this meant that she would only ask for me when I was working, which kept me pretty busy. But what I learned from this was that all people are not the same, their needs were not the same. And I started to see what they must feel living in these rooms, some without any visitors. The staff was their family. It was lonely and scary and they craved attention. I gave it to them. I took longer passing my meds because of it and therefore was written up twice.

I think one of the things I struggled with most was that the staff just saw this as a job. They saw what inconvenienced them. They didn't see the patients as human beings who had their own struggles, which were of course, far worse than ours. All they needed was a little kindness and compassion. Sometimes it was just mouth care or a warm blanket and I would watch the staff get so annoyed and take their time to respond. I never understood this.

I remember being called into my supervisor's office. I was told that my job was not a social job, that I was required to pass the medications in a timely fashion and focus primarily on that. "Visiting hours was not meant for staff". That was the last day I went back to that place. I called and said I couldn't come back. I know I could have handled that better. I had to fill out some exit paperwork after that and was very honest. I felt that their facility was clean, relatively organized and the residents/patients were for the most part in good care. My reason for leaving was that I wanted to do more and this was not the facility for me, for that type of care. I expressed a desire to treat them like humans, with feelings and respect their needs personally as well as physically. I was honest that I struggled with call bells not being answered or people sitting in wheelchairs for hours at a time in an empty lunchroom… and I went on. They actually called and asked me back several times after that. I have since heard that many things have changed for the better at that facility.

It was then when I knew without a doubt that I wanted to be a Hospice Nurse. I wanted to sit at the patient's bedside and comfort them. I wanted to make sure they were not alone.

Abruptly quitting my job was not the smartest thing I have ever done but it was the right thing for me personally. I was nervous about what I was going to do. I did not have a job lined up. But I absolutely could not work in that place any longer.

A few days later, a gal I went to nursing school with (the first time) called me up and suggested I apply at the company she worked for. She was one of the two people I thought of as "friends" during my first round of nursing school. We had issues, we were not always friendly towards one another, but we always respected one another as nurses and I never hesitated thinking about working with her professionally. She was a good nurse!! At the time they were in the process of purchasing a Hospice House and I was hired to work at the house when it became ready. Until then I would do home visits. The first year I was with this company, I visited patients in their homes. Most were elderly, some needed medication refills or wound care, some were bed bound, some could still walk and some were close to death and I was at their bedside when they passed away.

I remember the first time I knocked on a patient's door. I loved saying "Hi. I am your nurse". I loved being able to answer their questions, calm their fears and remind them that they matter and their thoughts and concerns were valid and deserved to be heard. Some patients I only saw one time, some patients I visited for several weeks, each one teaching me something and helping me to feel more and more confident in my ability as a nurse.

Some patients were cranky, some patients were rude, and some wouldn't even look me in the eyes.
Some were lovely, kind and appreciative.
Some talked non-stop.
Some didn't, or couldn't say a word.
Some lived in big houses, some lived in smaller spaces, one even lived outside in the garage.
Some spoke English, some didn't.
Some couldn't hear.
Some couldn't see.
Some couldn't walk or stand and one didn't have legs.
Some were scarred, some were bruised, some were bleeding, and most had pain.
Many offered me food, coffee or water.
Some had their family or friends nearby; some were all alone.
Each patient touched me.
Each patient taught me.
Each patient brought something into my life inspiring me to become the nurse I am now. I owe it all to them.

I gave my whole heart with each and every one of them. I opened myself up to them, sharing bits and pieces of who I am and how I came to be.

I listened.
I learned.
I loved.
I laughed.
I cried.
I found strength and I found struggle.
I realized my strengths and my weaknesses.

This experience was some of my best in learning my nursing skills. I started initially shadowing the gal I went to school with. She was a good teacher. She was very encouraging towards me and we worked really well together. Our supervisor was also very huge in my growth. She encouraged and supported me constantly and eased my fears when I was nervous about doing a procedure I was not completely confident about. All of this was growth for me. All of this was what gave me confidence as a nurse.

The next pages are stories of patients that climbed into my heart and found a permanent place there. You may need tissue.

Each family was approached and asked for permission. Those phone calls were beautiful, because we were able to reconnect for those few minutes and remember. I shared with each of them a quote I really love: "My memory loves you; it asks about you all the time". And for those few moments over the phone, we remembered. There were tears, lots of tears.

Nanny's Last Bath

My very first death pronouncement was for a family I didn't know and for a patient I had never seen before. It was out in a rural area, which was not well lit and the addresses were hard to see. I had to make several calls to the family asking for help with finding their home. I was flustered, embarrassed and nervous.

It was about 2am and although late, the entire family was up. They were tearful of course and her husband was so incredibly sad. They brought me to her bed; she was curled up like a small child with a beautiful green velvet blanket wrapped around her. I mentioned how pretty the blanket was, and her husband said, "It was her favorite". And he started to cry. Again. One of the younger kids came over and hugged him and all started to cry again. There was a lot of love in this house.

As we stood around the bed, I felt as though there was still more closure needed so I asked if they wanted to help me bathe her. I gave everyone a "job". Her husband went and filled a bowl with warm water and her grand children gathered washcloths and towels. I asked his daughter to pick out something we could dress her in. There was kindness in their energy as they prepared everything for what his granddaughter referred to as "Nanny's last bath".

While we bathed her, he told me about their life together. Theirs was a "beautiful dance of love" he called it. He shared that they met 65 years earlier at swing dancing class. Although he didn't tell her this for quite some time after their meeting, he only took the class because he saw her walk into the studio and wanted to meet her. He was eating lunch next door at the café; he watched her walk across the street and he remembered this joyful "bounce" in her step. He wanted to meet her, he knew at that first sighting that she was special. So he walked into the dance studio shortly after her, realizing there were classes about to start. The gal behind the counter asked if he was signed up for the class, he said no, so she encouraged him to sign up. He said "no" a few times but then she suggested he take the class once for free and if he liked it, he could buy a package for multiple classes. So he did. They were not partnered up until almost the end of the class. They danced well together. As they were leaving the dance floor she said to him "I hope we get paired up again at the next class". He giggled when he said, "Needless to say, I bought the package". He finally asked her out after about 5 classes and by then they became pretty good partners and as he said it, they have "been dancing together ever since".

Once bathed, we dressed her in the clothes her daughter chose. I found myself tearing up as she brushed her mom's hair. They were all so gentle and respectful with her.

As we waited for her to be picked up by the mortuary, I sat with the family as they continued to share stories. There was laughter and there were tears but most of all, there was so much love. Although my first, it still remains my most memorable.

A personal invitation

One day I was asked to visit a patient for another nurse because she was unable to see him. When I arrived, I was directed through the house to the family room, where the couch and coffee table were replaced with a hospital bed and side table.

We connected immediately. Our conversation went from the SF Giants, to 60's music, to the reason he doesn't eat chicken. We talked about his pain, his discomfort and the wound on his toe that wouldn't heal. And we talked about death. He was prepared for and accepting that he would be dying soon. All he wanted was to not be in pain.

I decided to tackle the toe first as wound care had become a passion of mine since I started nursing school. Within a week of treating the toe wound, it closed up. I am pretty sure that was the day his respect for me began. He started to open up to me about his thoughts on death and dying. Our conversations were deep, honest and thoughtful. I was invited into their family and became close with his wife and her daughter and together we gathered around him each day as he declined.

A few days before he passed away he called a meeting with the doctor, his wife and daughter, his Rabbi and myself. He said that he wanted each of us there when he passes. It was such an honor to be invited to be present at such a personal and intimate time. I also felt a sudden surge of selfish sadness at the thought of him leaving me. It's these moments that I am reminded it is not about me, but that is a difficult lesson to be mindful of. I find myself reeling my thoughts back in and focusing on what really matters; which is providing this man, this wonderfully kind man, the most peaceful passing I can. And at the same time provide comfort and support to his wife, who although very aware of what is happening, is still struggling with the thought of saying goodbye to her husband.

The day before he passed away I received a call from his wife; actually several calls. The first two were reassuring her that what he was experiencing was normal as he transitions. But she was scared and unsure and struggling with what to do and what her role was. I offered to come there. His wife, her daughter and myself were all gathered around his bed as he said his goodbyes to each of us. It was tearful and lovely all at the same time. It was getting late so I encouraged his wife to head to bed and her daughter to go home to her family. I promised to stay at his bedside, monitor him and administer the scheduled medications. I curled up in a chair next to his bed and every two hours I administered the medication and watched his breathing.

There is something incredibly peaceful sitting next to the bedside of someone who is actively dying on their terms. If I noticed his breathing change, I would reach out and touch his hand and remind him that I was there…and his breathing calmed.

The next day, his wife and daughter and I stayed at his bedside. His breathing started to change and his vital signs slowed. He was actively dying. We each told him it was okay to go, that we would all be okay and that we loved him. At that moment I felt as though I had known him all my life. I felt like a part of the family. I felt chosen and blessed to be at his bedside. The three of us women surrounded this wonderful man and took hold of each other's hands. We each cried. We sat in silence until he took his last breath. His wife crawled into the bed next to him and said goodbye. She thanked him for their life together and promised to love him forever. After about fifteen minutes, she got out of the bed and we each hugged one another. It was beautiful.

I remember leaving their house that day feeling so emotionally drained. I got in my car and I just cried. I was physically exhausted from so little sleep. I was emotionally drained from the entire experience, but I was also grieving my own personal loss. I liked this man, a lot. In the very short time we had together, we shared more than some share in an entire lifetime. To have someone trust you with their death is a responsibility like no other; an honor for sure, but such a deep commitment to someone else's very personal experience; one you cannot take lightly or only commit to half way. To be fully present for someone when they are dying mean's putting yourself aside and giving completely, being fully present and honoring their wishes the best that you can. I feel confident that I honored his wishes.

I am thankful that I have been able to stay in contact with his wife and daughter; we exchange messages frequently and try to get together for dinners. It doesn't happen with every patient, but sometimes I am blessed to take away a lifelong friend ship. This was one of those times.

Coloring outside of the lines

I started seeing a woman who had tumors on her lungs. Fluid was building around her chest cavity and pain was her main struggle. My job as her nurse was to drain the fluid from her lungs. This process took about an hour in total each time, which allowed us time to talk and get to know one another. She was an artist but had not been able to paint since she became ill. I was just starting out learning to paint using acrylic. She encouraged me to bring my paintings when we visited and shared her opinions very honestly. She told me often that I needed to go outside my norm, to color outside the lines. She talked about how she sees color and what inspires her to paint. She encouraged me to look at trees and flowers, the ocean, the sun, the moon… the sky. She taught me to see the colors in everything and when something strikes me, to pick up the paint and play. And I did.

She talked often about a trip she took years before, walking The Camino in Spain. We talked a lot about her experience on that trip and how much she learned about herself, and how much she grew. She constantly tried to talk me into booking the trip and doing it myself. She continually tried to push me out of my comfort zone; to try new things, to challenge myself, to break free and explore.

Our conversations were honest, creative, and full. We talked often about life and how fragile it can be. I tried everything to find ways to manage her medications in a way that would relieve her of pain. I made her smoothies and soups in hopes to entice her to eat. I called her every single day at 10am to check in on her. This became our routine. I did everything I could to help her find some semblance of comfort. I was not successful. She was in pain every single day. She had no desire to eat, and our visits always ended in tears. She decided to do the End of Life Option Act (EOLOA), which was about to become legal in California.

We spoke a lot about EOLOA in our visits. We talked about the conflict her family had with this decision. We talked about things she needed to take care of; the loose ends, the paperwork and the goodbyes. We talked about when and how and when, the "when" being the choice she struggled with most. Some days her pain was so bad, she wanted to do it that day. Some days it wasn't as bad so she thought she could wait a little longer. It was a constant tug and pull for her and I supported her every single day providing comfort, support and a listening ear.

She was finally ready, and set the date. She reached out to her Buddhist teacher to ask for prayer and support while she prepared herself.

She did not want many there but she wanted me there.

The day she was to do this, I arrived at her house. It was 4pm, in the middle of November so the sky got darker earlier. It was threatening rain. It took everything I had not to cry. I had been taking care of her for a year, she was my patient but she had also become my friend. I took a deep breath, walked in the door and I kissed her on the cheek hello. She was sitting in a chair, Indian style with a cup of tea in hand. She was so calm and peaceful. There were only a handful of people in the room as she was very selective in choosing who would be there that day. I met the doctor in the kitchen, where one by one each capsule was opened and spilled out into a small glass bowl.

As the medication went into the bowl, I said a tiny prayer for each capsule. "May her journey be safe", "may she know how loved she is", "may she never experience pain again". Each prayer was said with the intent to send her on her journey. My heart ached and yet at the same time I was so happy that this option had passed and people were finally allowed to make a decision to no longer suffer and to be able to die with dignity.

We finished preparing the medication and together, the doctor and I went into her room. We sat down and listened as the Buddhist prayers continued. When it was time, we walked over to her side of the bed. I kissed her on her cheek and said, "I love you." She said, "I love you too." She drank her medication and she sat crossed legged on her bed. In about 10 minutes, she looked over at me and said, "Wow, this is happening so fast. I am going now." And she waved goodbye and fell asleep. 30 minutes later she took her last breath; I said goodbye to my patient and my friend and she said goodbye to her pain and discomfort.

The next day her friend gave me a letter, which was left for me. She left all of her art supplies for me. As I loaded the brushes, the easel, the drawing pads, the paints and some of her paintings into my car, I cried. I already missed her. I drove home and brought everything into my tiny little studio. I started to scatter her things precariously around the room hoping it would fill with her energy, her light and her talent. That night I mixed some paints together, I put down the paintbrush and I swirled color around a blank canvas and I made magic happen. I watched as the paint played together creating a dynamic I could have never done with a brush. It was that day, that "Playing With Paint" was created and I started hanging and selling my paintings locally.

She inspired me in another way as well.
I booked the trip to Spain and I walked 200 miles alone along The Camino.
I thought of her every step of the way.

I think of her often. I am a better nurse because of the time I spent with her. She encouraged me to be brave, to be a little selfish and to embrace life and everything it has to offer and most of all to never settle for less than I deserve. Each time I create magic on canvas I send her a "thank you".

When I moved into my new house, she gave me some Buddhist prayer flags to hang outside. They are faded now; one even has a small rip. Sometimes I will look up at them and say hello to her and they will start flapping, with or without there being any wind. I know she is with me, I know she always will be.

The Hospice House – The people, the place, the heart

The Hospice House opened in October 2015 and I became a full time staff member. We had 10 beds with patients all within the last 2 weeks of their lives. Suddenly I was 100% fully dedicated to the end of life.

One of the first things I learned was that I am not a solo act. I do not do this alone and I couldn't possibly do it without the team of people I continue to be inspired by. Each person on staff brings a unique gift; each one a uniquely patterned fabric square that becomes the quilt of comfort for every patient that comes through our doors. We absolutely must work together, we absolutely must trust one another and we absolutely must encourage, and support one another, otherwise we cannot do what we do, as well as we do it..

I think one of the best lessons I learned, and still continue to learn in this process, is how to be a part of a team. The first mistake you can make in this business is thinking you know everything and assuming you can do it on your own. Our team was made up of the co-directors, medical doctors, case managers, spiritual support, social work, nurses, bereavement and grief support, home health aids and volunteers. Each member of this team contributes something valuable and it is up to you to find a way to work with them. You must truly understand what their role is and what they contribute to the patient, the families and your team.

I can't even count how many times I sat around a table with them and listened as they shared their thoughts, concerns, opinions and many times tears about a patient who was going through their process or whom had just passed. What I started to realize as time went on, was how incredibly valuable each of them were and how much I could learn from them. I started to get out of my own head and truly listened when they each spoke because I finally got it that I was going to be a better nurse because of each one of them. The more I listened the more I learned.

I could probably write an entire book just about this team. Each one has contributed to the nurse I am today and I will be forever grateful for the time they took to share their knowledge and experience with me. I appreciate their patience with me while I learned how to be a better team player. I appreciate their encouragement and support. I appreciate their kindness, compassion and unselfish hearts. Most of all, I appreciate them for inviting me into their space and making me feel so incredibly welcome even on my own worst days.

Sometimes when you first meet a patient and you stay at their bedside, you can't help but think of them as "your" patient and it is easy to become almost territorial. It is easy to think you know them best, or what their needs are, more so than anyone else. But this is far from true. In fact, what I have come to know is that I need the input from the team, I think everyone needs to hear what each other has to say.

Not all patients affect you the same. Not all climb into your heart permanently. The commitment to the care you provide is the same; the dedication and commitment to them is the same. But the affect they have on you is always different. When they pass away, you are grateful it was peaceful and you wish the family and loved ones comfort and strength, you hug yourself a bit and then you let them go. But sometimes you get a patient who for whatever reason touches you. Sometimes it is simply the way they look at you, or the way your touch provides them comfort, and sometimes it is because their presence reminds you of someone you might have lost. It doesn't matter whether you are with them a few hours, a few days or a few weeks, it's that moment you know you have just connected with them. A bond is formed and you have shared your heart and they have trusted you with theirs.

I am a crier. I cry easily and often. Anyone who knows me knows this. I don't always cry at every death though. And sometimes I don't cry for the patient, I cry for the pain and sadness I see from the loved ones left behind.

My pain is real.
My sadness is real.

One of the other benefits to having a team to work with is counting on them for support when you find yourself struggling with the loss of a patient. One of the things I have learned in this business is that rarely will your friends and family ask you how your day was; because most of the time... they don't want to know. I talk about death, a lot, and most people really struggle with hearing about it. It is really important to have an outlet, a release and someone to talk to. If you can find a partner that gets what you do, listens to your stories and comforts you when you struggle, HOLD ON TO THEM! TIGHTLY! The same goes for friends and family. Don't overwhelm them with the really emotional experiences but allow them to be there for you if they offer. Most people have no idea what a gift they are giving by just being there for us. I thank those of you who lend an ear, wipe a tear and give the big bear hug. Thank you!!!

There have been many days I really wish someone asked me how my day was, some days I just need a hug to help me get through my own personal grief when someone passes.

Not being overly spiritual most of my life and not having a commitment to a particular religion, I found myself quite surprised when the support I received the most comfort from was our spiritual counselors.

The first person I really started going to when I needed support for my own grief was the Buddhist spiritual counselor for our company. We connected immediately. Her presence was calming for me. Somehow she always knew when I needed her and she would send me a message "wanna go for a walk?" I would say "yes" and she would come find me. We would walk around the block a bit while I shared my grief; I would cry, I would let go and she would listen, share some wisdom or sometimes say nothing at all, just hold my hand and walk in silence down the street. I grew to really rely on her and we became friends. She continues to be a very calming force in my life and I am truly grateful for her.

Our Chaplain in the hospice house was always there for me with a hug or an ear when a patient passed that he knew I had grown quite fond of. He always seemed to know that moment when I needed him and he was always there. He started inviting our team into the patient rooms after they were picked up to say a prayer for them, to send them on their way with gentle words and to gather as a team to comfort one another.

Because of him I really started to embrace the commitment people have to their spiritual practice. I began to appreciate the power of prayer and faith. I appreciated his role in that of a patient who wants to pray, but more so for those who never did and at their last moments ask for some spiritual support.

My Aunt is a nun and while I never truly appreciated her commitment to her faith growing up, she has become a huge source of comfort for me. In fact I believe it is this job that I do which has brought us closer. Our conversations are deep, personal and incredibly honest. She has never judged me; in fact she is one of my biggest supporters. When she tells me she prays for me, I feel honored. I can talk to her about anything and her perspective has become very valuable to me. She has been at the bedside of the sisters as they pass, and knows probably more than most, how to be fully present for them. I have learned so much from her. I respect her commitment to her faith, but more than that I respect how open she is to what others believe in. I love how she has encouraged me to find my own path and has accepted me for who I am. We talk about death and we talk about life. I feel incredibly blessed to have her at my side.

With this profession, I have experienced many cultures and many faiths. I have watched people pray, sing, chant and read bibles. I have seen Rosary beads wrapped around hands, intertwined in fingers and laid gently across the chest. I have heard singing so loud the walls felt like they were shaking. I have seen crosses made of stone, brass, copper, silver and gold.

One time a Buddhist family invited three monks to sit inside the patient's room for hours chanting. I stood outside the door just listening and soaking it all in as I waited for them to call me in if needed. I was invited in periodically to check on the patient, thankfully able to calm him and relieve him of distress. When the Monks were finished they called me back into the room and asked if they could pray for me. I said yes. They tied a red string around my wrist and as they tied the multiple knots, they chanted. I felt blessed to be in their presence and I kept that string on my wrist until it fell off. Sometimes after that day, I would touch it and just close my eyes for a moment in hopes I could get brought back to that day when I felt so at peace.

There was a Baptist family that came, so many of them that they filled the entire living room of the house. And they would sing and play the piano and raise their hands to the roof as if to ask their God to please make sure her journey is safe and gentle. It was so incredibly powerful and I found myself in tears to see such love for their family and their God.

With strong faith comes comfort. To believe so strongly and have such commitment is powerful. I found strength in their strength.

I remember one of my first deaths at the house. He was so young; with a young daughter and a family so huge they overflowed the house out into the yard. They never accepted that he was imminent. They had faith and hope that he would survive. As a nurse I knew; I knew that he was close but they needed to hold onto whatever ounce of hope they had and I encouraged this. His brother was staying strong for everyone else but broke down with me in the office. He didn't want his brother to die; he didn't want his daughter to lose her father. Their heartbreak was deep and real and the bond between them all was beautiful. They called me into his room because his breathing changed. I went in and I knew. I knew he was close. I looked at his brother and he shook his head "no" as if to say "don't say it, do not tell us he is going to die". They were all gathered around his bed, looking at me for answers, answers I couldn't give. They asked me what to do. I looked at all of their faces and I knew at that moment I needed to give them something to do something to make them feel as though they did everything they possibly could for him. So I told them to pray. I told them to pray so loud the stars would hear them. I walked around the bed touching each one and yelling at them to pray louder. They prayed, and they prayed and he died. I waited a moment before I told them, I felt that they needed to finish. I looked at his brother and I shook my head "yes" and he knew. And he hushed the family; he told them God took him. It was peaceful, it was quiet and it was without struggle. His death was a beautiful death. I told them it was because of their prayers. They needed to know that and I believed it to be true.

    I was invited to the funeral; there were hundreds of people there. His brother got up and spoke. He talked about his illness and he talked about his death. And he mentioned me. He pointed me out for everyone to see me standing there. And he said "thank you". My heart was very touched that day.

    I have come to realize that most people have a very dark and scary opinion of death. The team of people I was lucky enough to work with were of the same mind; that death can be beautiful, peaceful, gentle and kind. Our job was to help to make that happen, but to also help the families believe it was possible. To relieve them of their fears and educate them through the process so they can be at the bedside and make a difference in the end.

    One of my favorite stories is of a brother and sister who did not communicate well, were not close and were hurtful to one another. When their father became ill and he was put on Hospice, they needed to make a decision on what the next step would be. Neither lived close to him, each living on opposite sides of the country, so bringing him to the Hospice House made most sense. His daughter was on board, His son was not; he was angry, aggressive and threatening a lawsuit. We see conflict and disconnect often, but this was by far the most difficult situation we had experienced. When one would come into his room, the other would leave. They did not speak to one another. The son questioned everything we did. The dynamic was difficult for the staff. Our team spent time with them individually, providing comfort and support, listening to them and assuring them that we would take very good care of their father. By the third day the son started thanking us for the care we provided, he brought us cookies and told us how grateful he was that he was there. He and his sister started talking. We provided them the safe place they needed to let their guard down, let go of their anger and come together. We encouraged them to eat together in the dining area and promised to stay at their dad's bedside while they ate. They started to sit in their dad's room together, one on either side of the bed using words like "we" when discussing his care and what "they" wanted for him. The last morning he was with us, his son went out to get lunch and brought it back for him and his sister. They ate together while we sat with him. We knew he was close, I think they did too. They decided to go for a walk and asked us to call if anything changed. A few hours later we made the call. They had decided to take a drive to the coast and hike along the beach. While they were out there, just before we called them, they said they knew it was time and sat on the sand and cried together, holding one another. They came back to the house and sat next to his bed. After he was picked up, they left together but not before thanking us for everything we did. We helped their father, but we helped them too.

Family dynamics are very common. By choice they avoid one another and some family members can go months or years without talking; but when someone is close to death they are almost forced to come together in the same space and be present. This is not an easy task. I think the difference between a home death and a facility death in these cases, is that the location is safe for both parties. It isn't one person's home that the other wants to avoid. Additionally we have experienced and trained staff to work with them, support them and listen to them. Best-case scenario is they come together and get past their difficulties. Unfortunately that is not usually how it works out. We do tend to act as mediators, sometimes buffers, and we relay messages back and forth. We will do whatever we can to alleviate some of the negative energy that drama can bring to the patient during their last days.

I remember this group of sisters of a gentleman who only had a few days left. This was probably the most disconnect I had ever seen between siblings. They were verbally abusive towards one another, each trying to draw our staff on their side. It was exhausting. They complained about one another, they each felt they were the better caregiver for their brother and picked apart the care, or lack there of, that the others did or didn't do for him. A few hours before their brother passed away they were arguing in his room; it was so loud I could hear it down the hall. I went into the room and asked if I could speak to them outside. Surprisingly they came with me. I admit I raised my voice, I even talked to them like badly behaved children but I also reminded them that their brother was dying and this was the very last time any of them would EVER see him alive again and they needed to really think about this last memory and whether or not THIS was how they wanted to remember this day. I asked them to stop this bickering and meanness; at least in front of him. I told them that I believe he can hear everything they were saying and asked them if these were truly the last words they wanted him to hear. I told them that I am sure he knows they wont be best friends and after this day, he probably also knows they will never talk again, but at the very least, give him the respect he deserves and tell him you love him, tell him you will miss him, tell him you will be okay and tell him goodbye.

They all went in there and did just as I suggested. Their brother passed away shortly after. There were a lot of tears and even some hugs. Two of the sisters left immediately. The other two stayed until he was picked up. As the sisters were leaving, one of them said "thank you" and hugged me.

Death is difficult. It is emotional. It is heavy and hard and brings out the very best in us but many times, the very worst. And this is normal. I go back to what I said earlier in this book, that one of the biggest lessons you learn in hospice, is that this is not about you. So when I am in a situation that I do not agree with or support or have a strong opinion about, I have to remind myself each time not to voice my opinion. But sometimes, you have to say something. Sometimes you have to remind someone else that this is not about them. And most times it is heard and responded to well.

The End of Life Option Act (EOLOA) is a very good example of that; as is palliative sedation, or choosing not to eat, or asking to have life-sustaining machines turned off or treatments discontinued. I have seen hundreds of people struggle from a diagnosis that is taking their life; I have seen that same amount of people take their last breath. And if I have learned anything at all, it is that all people have the right to choose. We do not have the right to judge, condemn or criticize the choices someone else makes for themselves; and in my opinion, especially relative to death. We may not understand it. We may not like it. It might not be something we would ever do. But that is THEIR choice. I also respect those that don't agree with these choices. I respect their personal opinions and beliefs. But again, I have seen a lot of death and if put in a situation like that I want to make sure I have a choice to not have my pain or suffering linger. I do not want to be hooked up to machines. I do not want medicines to prolong the inevitable. I don't want my family to sit at my bedside day after day, week after week or worse... months or years as I lay there struggling to live. That is not a good quality of life. My ultimate choice would be to have the opportunity to say goodbye, throw myself a huge party, dress up and look my best and go out with a bang. And after everyone leaves, swallow a half glass of water, mixed with EOLOA medications and close my eyes gently and peacefully. I want to have the choice to die with dignity and grace.

I have had many conversations with family members who are angry because their loved one stopped treatment, or stopped eating, or qualified for the EOLOA. And I had the same conversation each time; reminding them that this isn't about them. I try putting them in the patient's situation; I help them to envision the pain and the struggle. I remind them about having to be bathed or changed by someone else, sometimes sitting in their own urine or feces because they cannot verbalize that they are dirty. Or laying in a bed hearing other people talk about them, or listening to music they don't like on the radio because someone else chose it for them. Or laying there freezing because someone else thought it was too hot in the room, or placed a heavy blanket on them because someone else thought they were cold. That is not the life anyone wants to live. So if someone you love makes a choice like that, the very best thing we can do is support them, love them, and be there for them every step of the way because they are brave for making that choice and they deserve our love and support.

Most times, these conversations go over very well. Most times I am able to ease that person a little more towards providing comfort and support and further away from judgment and disapproval. I do not expect to change anyone's mind about anything. I respect everyone's right to choose; I will not judge you for who you vote for, pray to, kiss or what life/death choices you might make. But when I have a patient in my care, and they are dying, I will defend them, support them, protect them and advocate for them always.

I had a phone conversation with the friend of a woman who was riddled in pain for several years. She had multiple diagnoses and spent the past 5 years living life for those around her. She admittedly attempted suicide and was judged and punished by her family for it. Both times were unsuccessful. She chose to stop eating completely because in her option, she felt that was natural and neither God nor her family could judge this death. These were her words, not mine. And yet they did. They did judge her because they saw this too as "giving up" and as a form of suicide. I spoke multiple times with her friend. Finally, a few days before she passed away, I had the "this isn't about you" conversation and reminded him what life has been like for her all of these years. I helped him to see life from her eyes. And for the first time, it all made sense to him. He got it. And he felt guilty because he knew he had just wasted all these months being angry at her when what he should have been doing is loving and supporting her. He asked me to give her a message. He asked me to tell her he loves her. He asked her to forgive him for being so selfish. He asked me to tell her that he understands now why she needed to do what she did and he is okay with it, he understands it and he supports her decision. He said to finish with "I love you very much and I will miss you". I told her everything he said at a moment I felt she was alert enough to truly hear it. She opened her eyes, she said his name and she smiled. She was also tearful. I called him afterwards and let him know. I knew at that moment there was calm in both their hearts.

Anger, disapproval, unkind words or actions are like a very heavy blanket, one that is very difficult to remove. One of the best gifts you can give a person who is dying or to someone who will be left behind is forgiveness. Let them know you are sorry. Forgive them for whatever might be weighing them down. But more importantly, don't let that stuff linger when you have a full life to live. There are no do-overs. You only have right now, why waste it on meanness and anger and judgment and hurt? I ask people this question often: If you were to die today, is there someone you owe an apology to? Is there something you wish you should have or could have said? Is there a lie you need to provide truth for? Is there forgiveness you need from someone or need to give to someone? What if you did it now? What if you let it go now? What if you fixed it now? Imagine what a relief it would be for you and for them. Consider that.

I worked at the Hospice House for 2 years. It was the best experience of my nursing career so far. I grew as a human on so many different levels. And it was because of the team, the patients, the families and the staff.

I cannot say enough about the staff. I think the people that receive the least amount of credit for what they do, are the caregivers, the CNA's and the HHA's. These members of the care team are more up close and personal with the patients than anyone else. They bathe them, they change them and they feed them. They are with the patients at their most vulnerable of times. Losing your independence is very difficult; having someone else change you is degrading to many. And yet I have seen some of the most gentle, kind and compassionate hands on those members of our team. In most cases, whether it is a few hours, a few days or a few weeks, these patients become family members to the staff and that is how they are treated. If I can give any advice relative to them, it is to show them respect, appreciation and support. Thank them for the beautiful work they do. Support them when a patient passes because they feel this loss too, sometimes more than anyone else. I know this grief. I felt it when I lost the two patients I cared for when I was a CNA, before I became a nurse. I felt love and I felt loss. To be honest, I would be a far better CNA now, after seeing the work the team I worked with did. I wish I could have been more like them. Some of them have two or three other jobs; they can't possibly be getting enough sleep. Some of them support multiple family members, some of which who are out of this country. They should be applauded for the work they do.

There is a saying I seem to come across often:
"Be kind. For everyone you meet might be fighting a battle you know nothing about"

I think if we all really took to heart these words, we might treat each other kinder, we might show respect to others in a way we have lost site of and maybe, we would be just a little more aware of the difference a smile or a random act of kindness might provide to someone else.

I think of volunteers when I read my last words. In the Hospice House I was blessed to work with many volunteers. These are men and women of all different ages ranging from their early 20's to late 80's who volunteer their time to sit with patients or assist the staff in any way they might need. They are not there for payment, not even for compliment or recognition, in fact most shy away from that when we tell them how wonderful they are. They are unselfish, compassionate and kind and they are part of the beautiful quilt that makes up our team. Some read books to patients, some pray, some sing, some watch sports, some bring cookies or teas, some helped bathe or feed and some simply sat still being fully present as they transitioned and until they passed. I've hugged them, I've laughed with them, I cried with them and I grew to love them. They are beautiful, wonderful people who I admire and appreciate.

The Hospice House was a safe place for families to be able to let go of the physical responsibilities of caring for their loved one and hand it over to all of us so that they could be fully present. Most came to us with no idea what to do. For me I think this was the most rewarding part of my job. Seeing a friend or family member at the bedside struggling with finding the right words to say, draws me in. I truly loved being able to sit down with someone and help him or her to connect on a deeper level with the person in that bed. I educated people about death, about the process and what they are experiencing. I helped them to find something they could do that would provide comfort. Something as simple as rubbing a piece of ice on the inside of the wrist can cool them down; when I see a loved one doing this and watching their face when they realize they cooled them down, makes me smile inside. The unknown is very scary; most people do not know what death is like, they don't understand the process or the signs to look out for, or what to expect. I can't even count how many times someone has asked me "how long?" Death is very rarely predictable. When they have come to us, we understand it is inevitable but to tell someone a day or time is not possible. We can say, "they are close" or "it will be soon", and sometimes we are even able to get them all together minutes before the last breath is taken but we cannot always know. I have seen families think they have days and their loved one passes within hours of their arrival to us. I have also seen patients who were told they have hours but last days, weeks and even months. I have also seen a few go home because they ended up rallying and weren't quite ready yet. Those days are rare but wonderful. Some of those who went home also came back and we were able to be there for them when it truly was time.

Dying is very hard work. I feel like I have been taught by and have worked with the best teachers. I have learned how to put aside vital signs and medical terminology and truly see what that person is experiencing and find ways to reduce their struggle. While I do feel medication is necessary and in most cases, a peaceful death requires it, I also believe in tactile stimuli and the comfort of human touch. There is so much fear surrounding death; both from the patient and those who love them. I focus on reducing fear. I encourage handholding. I encourage touch. I encourage words. All of these things help reduce fear.

Swishers

She came to us with only a few days left to live. She was rough around the edges, she had a trucker mouth and she was feisty. I loved her immediately. She had uncontrollable pain, she was uncomfortable and she was really pissed off about it all. We helped manage her pain and each one of us took turns trying to reach her. I think I won!

Her husband visited her every morning before work and every night after work. Some days were good, some days were bad and it was difficult to watch how hard this was on him. But he never stopped being there for her. Some days she ignored him, some days she yelled at him, some days she slept through his visit, and most days, she cried after he left, because the truth was, that she didn't really want him to go. Pain was her main symptom, but knowing you were dying but not knowing when was torture for her. Her days turned into weeks and soon her friends and family stopped coming by. She was very devastated by that.

She subscribed to multiple magazines so one day her husband brought in about 20 of them. He joked about how she was sure she was going to win Publisher's Clearing House one day, so she subscribed to every magazine she could. He told many funny stories about her and shared so many photos. Their relationship had its ups and downs, like most do, and they had survived many difficult times, but they survived them together.

She was a smoker that hadn't had a cigarette in awhile. She smoked grape "swishers" and talked about them often. So one day, I went out and bought her some. I asked her if she wanted to "break out of this place and smoke". She was so excited. We got her out of bed, we wrapped her up in blankets and I wheeled her out the door into the sunshine. This is a moment I will remember forever; because it was on this day that I was reminded just how much we take for granted. She looked up at the sky as though she'd never seen it. She breathed in the air with pure joy. She hadn't been outside in a very long time. I pushed her down the block towards the alley behind a bar that opens at 6am. It seemed fitting. We sat there in the alley and smoked a swisher. Together.

About two days later she declined significantly. She was no longer responsive and we knew she was close. Her husband stayed at her bedside and I rarely left it myself. About 6pm one night when I had gone home, he called me and asked if I could come back and sit with him. So I did. He sat on one side the bed and I sat on the other. Her breath changed and her hands became cold; I sat there and rubbed them continuously. He fell asleep and I sat next to her watching her breathe. She took one deep breath, as though she was breathing it all in, and then she passed away. I walked over to where he was sleeping and nudged him until he woke up. I whispered "she passed" and he started to cry. I left him alone with her for a bit.

When I came back in, I sat down next to him. I reached out for his hand and we sat in silence. He said, "I am going to miss her so much". He didn't stay and wait for her to be picked up. Not everyone does and that's okay. I promised I wouldn't leave her and that we would bathe her and escort her out when it was time.

A few of us went to the funeral; there were only a few people there. There were pictures of her from before she became ill; she was a very pretty woman. Her husband was nervous and awkward; socializing wasn't his thing. I think he found comfort by us being there. Their friends and family let them down those last few days by not really coming around so I have a feeling he will hold that grudge a long time.

Once a month for about a year he would come by the house and bring us magazines, he said he didn't have the heart to cancel the subscriptions. We talked about her and how much he missed her. His life would go on but it would never be the same.

On her year anniversary we spoke. I don't think a day will ever go by that he won't think of her. We have stayed in touch, we probably always will.

A promise kept

He came to us several months after we had provided end of life care for his daughter's friend. When he started to decline, his daughter came to us and asked us to take care of her father. We agreed immediately. I remember really liking her and thinking how bittersweet it was that we were seeing her again.

I remember seeing his name and thinking it was familiar. And then it hit me, he was one of my very first patients a few years prior when I was doing my clinical rotations. At that time he was up and about in a wheel chair bossing people around and being kind of grumpy. I liked him immediately. When he would see me walk in, he would turn his head as though he were hiding and pretended he didn't see me. I would walk up to him and say hello, he acted as though he didn't know me and I would reintroduce myself to him. It was a game we played. I would walk away and he would ask me to come back. The first day he was at our house and I saw him in the hospital bed, I was reminded that I never told him goodbye. I did my training at his facility for several months and then suddenly we were told to go somewhere else, so I never went back. I felt a sense of guilt as I sat at his bedside. I whispered in his ear that I promised to see him through this and make sure that he was well cared for, and loved. This was before I had the chance to meet, and fall madly in love with, his family. This promise was going to be an easy one to keep.

He was only with us a few days, but it seemed longer. I was given an opportunity to spend time with his incredible family. I felt like each one of his children brought a unique gift into my life. It was as though each one represented a part of me that I could relate to so easily within them. I could write pages about each one because they touched me that deeply. I was lucky enough to spend quality time with them, get to know them, hear their stories and share some of my own. His wife was surrounded by so much love, but her pain and sadness was deep. She didn't talk about it and she didn't express it, but I knew. I knew this was hard for her, I knew it would take a very long time for her to heal. Sometimes I would just sit next to her, sometimes I would take her hand, and sometimes I would just look at her and smile. And always I would cry.

I felt honored to be in the room one night as they all sat around his bed telling stories. There was so much laughter and so much love and so many memories. This family touched me. They supported one another, they protected and cared for their mom and they made sure that their dad was never alone. I made sure of that as well. I spent a lot of hours at his bedside that night, far after my shift ended. I found it hard to leave. I knew in my heart I had made him a private promise and I was not going to let him down, but it was more than that. I think I felt the need to be there for the family as well. I don't think they needed me, I think they would have been just fine if I wasn't there, but I needed to be there for him and for them. I was drawn to them, pulled into their circle and felt such safety and comfort and love that it was very difficult for me to leave. Could some say I crossed a line? Perhaps. Should I have left and gone home at the end of my shift? Maybe. There are so many things we can all say we should have done differently at one time or another, and while this might be one of them, I know without a doubt that my being there with them was exactly where I needed to be.

I wasn't there when he took his last breath. I didn't feel bad about that, which is a good thing. His family was there and our incredible staff was there, so I knew he was in good hands. But I was called and I immediately went in. The family had spent the past few days preparing for this moment so by the time I walked in, they were sad, understandably, but so strong and loving and accepting of his passing. They were able to take those days to embrace his life and prepare for his death. I walked into a loving family, supporting one another, hugging one another and laughing and feeling whatever it was they needed to feel. It was healthy, it was human and it was beautiful.

I asked them to stay and wait for him to be picked up. There was hesitation when I explained our rose petal ceremony, but I felt compelled to encourage them to be a part of it. I had a feeling this would be the gentle closure they needed and a beautiful goodbye for him. And it was.

They had a large family presence. As we all lined up to wait for him to be wheeled down the hall, their family went from one end of the house to the other. A bowl of rose petals was passed around and each one stood quietly as their fingers caressed the soft petals, waiting for him to come. As he came around the corner, we all sprinkled rose petals over him as he was pushed past us; each one of us saying goodbye; some in whisper, some with tears. And then we all gathered outside as he was loaded in the car and watched as he was driven away.

The family hugged one another and they hugged each of us, thanking us for the care we provided. What they don't know is what happened after they left. It took a little bit as they gathered their belongings, and cleaned up his room. Once they had all left, we gathered in a circle, holding hands in his room and stood quietly while we wished him a safe journey. Some prayed, some cried and I reminded the staff what a beautiful job they did for him and his family. We hugged one another and we continued on with our day.

About two weeks later I remember sitting in the dining room when the doorbell rang. I went to answer it but no one was there. This happened multiple times. Finally I just left the door open, assuming perhaps it was "someone" coming back. I think it was "him". So I sent a message to his son, hoping he wouldn't think I was totally whacky. As it turns out, something similar had happened with him as well, so he was sure it was his dad. Once I left the door open, the doorbell stopped ringing. I like to think that he came back to thank me for keeping my promise. Or maybe he wanted to be in the place his entire family had last gathered. Either way, I felt such peace knowing he was there. I went to the service and I have maintained a friendship with his children and his wife. They have my heart and they always will.

Wild Bill

Obviously that wasn't his real name, but it is what I called him, because that is what he told me to call him when we first met. He was in his late 80's when he came to us. Riddled in pain but never said a word to anyone about the depths of pain he was truly feeling. His family gathered around him and showered him with love. He was sweet. He was a flirt and wooed all the lady nurses; kissing our hands and smiling at us through his sparkling blue eyes.

His family was so full of love. His grandkids arrived, each in their late 20's and spent what they called "cuddle time", taking turns laying next to him in his hospital bed. They sang songs to him, they laughed with him and they told him many times how much they loved him.

He was a strong man, a man that would not reveal to anyone just how much pain he was in. I could see it though; every time he was repositioned, every time he was bathed or changed I could see in his face that he was fighting pain. I offered to give him something but he only ever wanted Tylenol. As a nurse, it is really tough knowing you can relieve someone of pain and having him or her resist. He was being so strong and brave and something we often see, is this obligation to not give the reason for the family to worry. He felt obligated to be the strong one.

I sat down with his daughter and explained that it was my opinion her father was in far more pain than he was saying and that I felt he needed more medication to relieve him of pain. She understood this but was more concerned with how her mother would feel and asked that I sit down with her and help her to see how much he had declined, that he was probably in a lot of pain and explain to her the medications we would like to try and help her to understand what to expect.

I invited her mother, his wife of 60 years, to sit with me on the couch. I took my time and was very careful with my words; I imagined myself in her position. 60 years married to the only man she ever loved was going to be a really tough thing to let go of. I told her that I felt he was in more pain than he was being honest about and she agreed. I took my time educating her on medication that by name usually make people very fearful. Medications are scary. Hearing words like "Morphine" tend to make people think we are ending someone's life. Most people do not know as much about the medications as we do, which is completely understandable. It is my job as their nurse to help them to feel safe, to educate them on any medication we might consider giving and to give them time to absorb all the information in such a way that they are no longer fearful and can feel confident that this truly is the best thing for him.

I explained two medications the doctor felt would reduce his pain and the anxiety from the pain. I told her they were friends and played nicely together. I explained how both, would bring him comfort. She asked if he would die. I explained that I could not predict that, but perhaps he is ready and the pain has been so intense he has not been able to relax and let go. I explained that he has not slept well in several days and these medications might allow him to finally sleep, and that yes, there was a possibility this would be the time he transitions and would pass peacefully. I wanted her to know all possible outcomes, to be completely prepared for whatever might happen in the coming hours. She was accepting of trying the pain medications.

I prepared the medications. I got a small bowl of chocolate ice cream and I went to his bedside. I told him what I was about to give him and why. I looked in those beautiful blue eyes and told him I didn't want him to be in any more pain. He took my hand, brought it close to his mouth and kissed it. He looked into my eyes and whispered "thank you". I gave him a bite of ice cream; I gave him his medication, followed by another bite of ice cream. I kissed him on his forehead and said "sleep peacefully Wild Bill… no more pain for you". And he smiled. I walked out of his room and I cried.

I cried because I could see he was grateful for what I did. I was his advocate and spoke for him when he couldn't do it for himself. I felt like a patient advocate in the truest sense of the word.

A few minutes later his daughter and granddaughter came to me and thanked me. We were each very tearful. Wild Bill slept a few hours without any signs of pain or distress. When he awoke he was rested and able to verbalize that "was the best sleep I've had in a long time". He was with us a few more days and when he did finally pass, it was peaceful and calm with his wife and daughter loving him at his bedside.

About a year after that, I ran into his wife and daughter. We spoke about that time a year before and they thanked me again for being honest with them in such a sensitive way. They were able to have time with him, to say goodbye and to be present for his death, which was peaceful.

I remember when I saw them, how happy my heart was to see them. I think they felt the same. No matter how much time passes, those moments you share with someone never go away. They are special memories, that although take you back to a difficult time, make you smile through the tears.

Wonder Woman

She was very young, too young to have a terminal illness. She was married and had a few young children. She was a wife and a mommy but too ill to be either any more and this broke her spirit. Despite this though, she always kept a smile on her face when her kids where visiting. She never let them see her cry.

She came to us because she was at home and her care required more than her family could provide and it was her choice to leave their home and come to our facility. She was one of the most unselfish people I have ever known.

She spent several weeks with us. She was partially paralyzed, which made it difficult for her to do anything on her own. She refused to ask for help initially because she didn't want to bother us; but we continued to remind her that we were here to help her and encouraged her to trust us. We left a bell at her bedside and asked her to ring it when she needed us. It took her quite some time to ring that bell… but when she finally felt comfortable with it… the ringing was constant. Sometimes I think she needed something but most times, I think she just didn't want to be alone.

She loved sliced peaches and Sponge Bob Square Pants.
She giggled like a small child when something pleased her.
She said "thank you" with her whole heart.
She let us all in and became very dependent on our presence, our support, our compassion and our care.

Her husband was strong and brave.
She was strong and brave.

Theirs was an incredibly sad situation that affected us all. I call her Wonder Woman because she was so strong and brave. She liked super heroes, something we had in common. She always put everyone ahead of herself. She fought her battle with grace, acceptance and strength, despite how much it broke her inside. I bought her a Wonder Woman cape, which she wore her last few days.

When she passed away, several of us assisted in bathing her. We cried during the process. I cry as I write this, because I remember how I felt that day. We lay the Wonder Woman cape across her chest. We played Amazing Grace as she was rolled out to the car and we sprinkled her with red rose petals. She has a permanent place in my heart. I promised her I would check in on her husband once in awhile. I have called him a few times. He is healing. He is strong. And he will be forever thankful for us, and the way we loved and cared for her, for him and for their kids.

Cherry Blossoms

This was a woman who touched every single person she met. She was gentle, she was kind, and she was lovelier than any human you will ever meet. And she was dying.

She was with us for several weeks. Her room was decorated in fairy lights her husband hung for her. There were cards on string that draped across the walls from friends. She considered them art and felt they were too beautiful to be kept in a drawer. There were pictures her students had drawn for her wishing her well and hoping for a recovery. There were Origami swans placed precariously around the room and crystals and healing beads on whatever tabletop space she could find. There was a feeling of hope that filled her room at all times; because despite the terminal diagnosis and the fact that we knew her time was short, no one wanted to believe it to be true and none of us acted as if it were. Especially her.

She drank teas and took herbal remedies hoping it would give her more time. She welcomed healing touch often and a visit from a Shaman, which provided her with a sense of calm and inner peace.

I was drawn to her. We had many beautiful, personal moments that I will cherish forever. She was an art teacher. She loved art, she was inspired by art and she encouraged others to tap into their creative side. I shared with her some of my paintings. She was always so supportive and complementary. I remember when I received the confirmation that I would be hanging my paintings in a restaurant. I was so excited. I told her about the "artist reception" that was being planned and I was so proud. The day before the reception, she asked me to come to her room. She handed me a rock that said, "imagine" on it and told me to start believing in myself, and to imagine that anything I wanted was possible. I kept that rock with me during the reception and I continue to touch it every morning as I start my day.

Every one of the staff loved her.
She loved every one of the staff.
I think she said, "I love you" to every person that walked in and out of her room, and she meant it and we felt it.

As she became weaker, we all knew it was getting closer. This was a day we hoped would never come but knew it eventually would. When she had the energy, she would make each person an Origami swan that was in his or her favorite color. She gave special books, or sentimental trinkets away to some, asking that they remember her always. I was a lucky recipient of one of her gifts; it was a hand carved floating dragonfly made of bamboo. It sits with my Origami swan and my rock that says, "imagine".

We filled her room with fresh cherry blossom branches in clear vases for her to see from her bed. We hung iridescent butterflies near the window, which moved gently back and forth. And we took turns sitting quietly at her bedside while she slept. Despite how weak she was, she would open her eyes, see one of us there and smile as she would say our name, followed by "I love you" and then fall back to sleep.

We reminded each shift, as we would leave, to call us if she was close, because every single one of us wanted to be there when she passed. We wanted to say our goodbyes, but more than that we each needed our own closure.

I remember the day she passed very well. It was in between the NOC shift and the AM shift and we were having endorsement. One of our home health aids came and said she was close. We dropped everything and each one of us circled around her bed, held hands and told her we loved her. I looked around at the staff and admired their beautiful hearts. There was so much love in that room. Each person kissed her cheek, told her they loved her, thanked her and said goodbye.

A few hours later, as a small group of us were at her bedside, she took her last few breaths and passed with grace, beauty and peace. She did not need any medications, she did not struggle; she embraced every last breath and she closed her eyes for the very last time.

We filled bowls with cherry blossoms and we scattered them on her as we all walked her out to the car. We cried. Sometimes we still cry just talking about her. Sometimes we feel her energy. She will never leave our hearts. She was that patient that touched each one of us and she was the piece of thread that connected all of our fabric pieces together. She helped secure our quilt. We are all better humans because of her.

Saying Goodbye

I arrived at a house of a patient I had never met. His daughter greeted me and asked to talk to me before introducing me to her father. She wanted to know what we could do to help him "come out of this". She was hoping food or IV fluids could revive him. She was tearful, she was stressed out, she was sad and she was fighting the reality that her father was dying.

She walked me down a long hallway to a room that was packed full with 70 years worth of memories. I had to climb over chairs and boxes to get to the side of the bed but even before reaching her dad, I knew. I knew he was very close and no amount of water or IV fluids could change that.

I sat down with her dad, visually assessed him and looked up at his daughter, who stared back at me with eyes that said, "do not tell me he is dying". She asked me what I thought. She asked me what I could do. She asked me how much time he had left. And in the same breath, she said, "he is dying isn't he"? I got up, I walked towards her and I reached out to hug her. She put her head on my shoulder and for a few moments, just stood crying.

We sat down outside for a bit and I explained the dying process. She wanted to know what she could do, how she could help her dad. I told her to be fully present for him, thank him for the gifts he brought into her life and tell him she would be okay. Give him permission to let go. She said they had a fight a few weeks ago and felt bad. I encouraged her to apologize, explain where she was coming from and ask for forgiveness. The one thing I truly believe is that no matter how unresponsive a person is, they can still hear you and feel your energy. What you say and how present you are during their last hours can absolutely affect the peacefulness of their passing. I believe this with all of my heart.

We went back inside and she crawled into the bed next to her father. She told him how much she loved him as she brushed his hair with her fingers. She talked about her childhood and thanked him for being such a good father, and forgave him for the days he wasn't. As she continued, I slowly got up and waved goodbye as I walked out the door.

She slept next to her father the entire night. When she woke up, she said her dad took one long, deep, last breath and passed away in her arms. She was fully present for him. She made this about him and for him. She was able to say "thank you", "I love you" and "goodbye".

Baby Doll

I received a call from one of our social workers asking if I could come see a patient. There was urgency in her voice as she indicated she wanted him seen soon. He was grumpy (for lack of a better word) and slightly difficult to work with. He had practically thrown out every member of his team that tried to visit him. She warned me this visit would be difficult.

When I arrived, I knew immediately it wasn't going to be easy but I love a challenge and was ready to take him on. He was a man in his 60's, too young to die, with only 3 months having to digest a terminal diagnosis and very little time left to live. Of course he was difficult, he was angry, really, really angry. I started off by asking him what he needed from me. And I listened to him; I really listened. When he was finished I understood that he needed his pain relieved, so I started there. I talked about different ways we could manage his pain, he let me know which route was the best for him and I called his doctor. A plan was initiated that night.

He was Italian with a big voice and a lot of hand movement. He was frustrated, impatient, sarcastic and very matter a fact. But he was also very sweet, and a bit of a softy and we bonded quickly. He was known for his Risotto; one night he sent me home with a big container of it. It was delicious.

I only had about 4 weeks with him. I saw him several times a week, I even saw him on Christmas morning. He called me often and I always responded. He trusted me. I earned his trust very quickly and I wasn't going to let him down.

He was a golfer, a pro to be exact. Golfing was his life. Whenever his put would roll in, he would say "baby doll" (hence the title of this story). It was a slogan he said often and something everyone connected him with. He refused to use a walker or a wheelchair, insisting on using his golf club for support until he could no longer walk. He did things his way and there was no arguing with him.

I met his girlfriend; they only just started dating when he was diagnosed. He gave her the option to step out of the relationship but she didn't. She was amazing. People call hospice nurses angels but I think its people like her who should have that title. She took wonderful care of him; she learned all his medications, she changed his dressings, she cleaned up vomit and dirty sheets, she held his hand, she stayed at his bedside and she told him she loved him, every single day. She was so incredibly lovely.

I met his son, who's heart shed light on everything around him. He was gentle and kind and sweet and sad, terribly sad. And he was good to his dad until the end. As was his mother. His sister, struggling with her own personal loss months earlier, rallied for her brother. Her grief still fresh, she truly struggled with everything her brother was experiencing and yet she was so fully present for him. She flew to be at his bedside and she advocated for his needs beautifully.

His decline happened quickly. His pain was aggressive and mean and I struggled to manage it. We tried everything we could but it just would not let up. With his pain also came nausea. As a nurse, it was difficult for me that I could not do more for him. I wanted so badly to give him more time, to give his son, his girlfriend, and his sister more time. And to be honest, I wanted more time with him too. I had hope and I encouraged hope but deep down inside I knew. His time was short.

One night about 10pm I received a call from him. He was crying. The pain and the nausea had broken him, he was done; I went to see him right away. He asked me to talk to the doctor about palliative sedation. It was decided that he would go to the hospice house because he required more care than his family or girlfriend could provide, despite their desire to.

Just before the ambulance came to transport him to the house, he requested his dark glasses and leather jacket. Once again doing things his way, on his terms, and with flair. I watched as he was wheeled out the door and I smiled because his dramatic exit was awesome, but I cried too because I knew he wasn't going to be with us much longer. We all knew this was the beginning of our goodbye.

Taking him to the hospice house was the best decision for so many different reasons. It allowed everyone to be at his bedside and fully present without having to do the difficult physical work. The wonderful staff bathed him, managed his medications, and provided care and comfort to the family. Palliative sedation was initiated. The family took turns at his bedside, saying their goodbyes and giving him permission to go. I stayed with them as much as I could.

He passed away two days later, peacefully, pain-free and with his girlfriend at his bedside holding his hand in hers. I went to the celebration of his life, which was at a golf course, in a room filled with golfers, all of who really liked this guy. I looked outside the window and all the golf carts were parked in one long line. I thought to myself; instead of the 10-gun salute, he received the 10-golf cart salute, which was not intentional but it was fitting.

He was a good, kind man and I am grateful to have had time with him. I am very fond of his family and his girlfriend. I think we will stay in contact for the rest of our lives. We only spent a few weeks together but the bond was immediate and tight.

One night I was at the bedside of a woman who only had a few hours left to live. Her daughter sat on the other side of the bed. Her mom was actively dying, and having a really tough time. I would reach over, place my hand over her heart and touch her very gently, letting her know that she was safe and she was not alone. Her breathing would calm and for a few moments, her process was peaceful. Her daughter watched me, but said nothing. I did this several times. I asked her if she would like to try it. She looked at me with uncertainty in her eyes. I explained that while I was probably bringing comfort, it would be her presence that would provide the most comfort for her mother and encouraged her to try it. She slowly placed her hand over her mother's chest when her breathing became rapid. She looked at me for guidance, I told her to go with her heart, trust herself. She placed her hand over her mother's heart and the breathing slowed. She whispered in her mother's ear and told her she loved her, that it was okay to go and that she would be right there by her side to comfort her. The look in her eyes when she watched the calm come over her mother was beautiful.

These are the things that inspire me most in my job. I have been present for more deaths than I can count and I do find true pleasure at the thought of being responsible for changing what could have been a difficult death, to one that is peaceful, and beautiful. But what brings me the most joy, is showing a loved one something they can do to bring peace to someone they love at the most difficult time of their life. I think it helps with their grieving process. There is a moment when I step away from the bed and allow a family member or a friend provide that role and it fills my heart, because I know it fills theirs too.

Medication is almost always necessary at the end of life, but tactile stimuli, true deep love and being completely present, provide something that medication can't touch. Some people want to be alone and some do not want their hands held or someone sitting at the bedside. But most do. Most want you to reach for their hand, tell them they are not alone and give them permission to go in peace.

I struggle when I walk into a room with someone who is about to die and there are family or friends sitting around the bed in total silence or on their phone or distracted by a television show. I believe they hear everything even after their last breath. They also feel everything; they feel your energy when your back is turned or you are distracted by something that has absolutely nothing to do with them. If they love music, play it for them. If you are at their bedside, talk to them. Tell them you love them and thank them for the gifts they brought into your life. Tell them you will be okay.

I am a nurse, I know what to do but not everyone else does, so I like to educate. I like to share the things I have learned and pass them on so someone else, who is closer and more intimate with the patient, so they can provide care that will forever impact their heart and make for a much smoother passing for someone they love.

Someone asked me what I hoped to achieve by writing this book. She asked me if there was a specific message I wanted to send out. What I realized while writing this book is that people are afraid of death. Death is scary and there is so much unknown. People don't know what to do or what to say. There is fear, a lot of fear. I think if I could achieve anything with this book, it would be to help people come out from under the dark cloud that floats all around death. Yes it is scary, it is emotional, it is painful and it sad. I have said that a few times in this book. Because those are all real and true; but death can also be peaceful, gentle, kind, safe and sometimes it can even be incredibly beautiful.

I had a patient when I first started working in Hospice, whose illness took a sudden decline very quickly. She could no longer get out of bed to use the bathroom and her husband and daughter had to help change her, and then caregivers had to be at her bedside at all times. This was not the way she wanted to spend her last days. She was riddled in pain; she knew she was going to die soon. She decided to start palliative sedation and die with some dignity and on her terms. When I heard this news, my heart ached. It was incredibly selfish of me, I know this, but I liked her, I liked her a lot and I was really struggling with saying goodbye.

A few days after she passed away, I went to see her husband and daughter. We talked about that last day. He had climbed into the bed next to her just before the medication was started. They were left alone in her room, given privacy to share their last few hours together before she slipped into a sedation that would finally end her pain. I asked him what they talked about, what their last words to one another were. I watched as his face took on the most beautiful smile with a look of so much love as he told me they lay there together in bed and told each other how much they love one another, they shared memories of things they did together and moments they shared. They did this until she closed her eyes and went to sleep. He will get to hold that memory in his heart for the rest of his life. Prior to her starting the palliative sedation, he said, "I thought we would have more time", but after she passed, he said he was so grateful because if it had happened any other way, he would never have had those moments, those memories, that goodbye and all that expression of love. She died on her terms; with her husband and daughter at her bedside. She died knowing how loved she was. It was a beautiful death; no distress, no pain, peaceful and completely on her terms.

This memory has stayed with me for several years; it continues to motivate me to do my part in helping each patient have a more peaceful death, a beautiful death, and a soft landing.

Your last words, whether they are at the bedside of someone dying, or when someone walks out the door on their way to work could very well be the last ones they hear from you. You don't get a do-over and you can't take them back. Think about that.

I received a call from the son of a patient who had just passed away the day before. He had a few questions about things someone else would need to help him with, but during the conversation I asked him how he was doing. He started to cry. He talked about his dad. I said, "it sounds like your dad was a very good dad" His son went on about the life his dad gave him, the lessons he taught him. He wanted more time with him. I hear that a lot.

His father was going to be cremated. He wanted to know if he could send something with his dad. "Sometimes people leave things in caskets before the burial, but how do you do that for someone who is cremated". He jokingly suggested tying a ribbon around his dad's toe. This invited an absolutely lovely conversation. I suggested he and his siblings each take a different colored ribbon and tie it around his toes, or his ankle or his wrist. Much like the Monks do with the red string, saying a prayer or a wish for a beautiful journey as each knot is tied. He loved this idea.

About a week after the cremation, the son called me. He and his siblings and their mother, together with their ribbons, each said something special to him as they tied the knots. He said it was beautiful. This made me smile.

I remember a wife of a patient asked that her husband be buried with his workout gloves and hat. After he passed away, I helped her bathe him and we dressed him as though he were going to the gym. She had brought a framed photo of him when he was healthy and working out regularly; such a strong and handsome man. It seemed fitting for him to be buried that way. After we dressed him, she placed the framed photo in his arms and we waited for the mortuary to come. When they got there, one of them reached for the frame to hand to his wife. She told them she wanted him to go with it. They did not question it; in fact they placed the photo back in his arms and were careful when they placed him on the gurney so that the photo would not fall. It was a gentle kindness that did not go unnoticed.

Grief

One of my most humbling realizations was learning to let go of my tools and hand them to the loved ones. Learning to step back was huge for me. It is so easy to step in and guide the family from the bedside but what I have come to realize is just how much better it is for the family if I give them the tools and teach them how to use them.

What I have noticed is that the grieving process is just a little gentler when the family is involved in the care, and when they are fully present at the bedside. I find such joy stepping back and watching them.

I hear people say "it will get better with time" after someone passes away. I struggle with those words. My sister passed away several years ago, she was sick for a very long time and she fought the good fight. After she died, I couldn't help thinking I wished I could have done more, visited more, told her in more depth the true effect she had on me all these years. I have regrets. And it has not gotten easier; in fact I think it has become more painful for me because I miss her terribly. When I was going through nursing school, she supported me from a hospital bed. She encouraged me every step of the way. She did this all my life as well; she was ALWAYS good to me, even when I did not reciprocate. I have learned that it does not get better with time. It gets a little less painful maybe. But loss is loss.

I think of grief as an ocean. Some days the waves come up gently against the shore, they linger there a bit and then slowly roll back to where they started. Some days though, it is like wild crashing waves coming down so hard on the shore it feels as though they could break something and when they go back out, it takes a little piece with you. But it can work the other way too. You can stand at the shore and as a wave comes toward you, ask it to please carry some of the pain you are feeling away, hand it to the ocean, ask it to help you. This works for me.

Death is emotional. Loss is emotional. Missing someone is painful. Death reminds us how beautiful life is and how much we take for granted. My advice to people after someone dies is to go through the emotions, whatever they may be. Cry when you need to. Feel everything as deeply as you need to. Don't hold anything back. But also, don't be afraid to laugh or smile. There will be moments where you might find something funny or you will be having a good time and you stop because you think you shouldn't be feeling this way or acting that way. Stop that. Laugh, play, and enjoy your life. The person you said goodbye to would want you to enjoy your life.

Life is fragile, it is unpredictable and there are no guarantees or promises that anything beyond this very second is for sure. And yet as humans we continually think beyond the tomorrows and we use words like "one day" when we talk about something we hope to do. If I have learned anything at all in my work, it is that right this very moment is the only thing we can be certain of. I have learned that you can never say, "I love you" too much. That sometimes a hug says so much more than words. And I have learned that kindness and compassion are the best gifts you can give someone else whether they are family, a friend or a complete stranger.

Death doesn't have a time clock, it doesn't know if it's day or night, Monday or Tuesday or whether it's a holiday or the Super Bowl. Death is not predictable. Because of this it is our responsibility to make sure that moments matter, that we make right now the very best that it can be.

Be good to one another.
Be kind. Be respectful. Be patient.
Embrace life.
Embrace love.
Embrace friendship.
Embrace family.

With so much love and gratitude to every single person who helped me along this journey, I say thank you. To my friends and family who supported me, to the patients and their families who trusted me, and to all of my teachers.... I became the nurse I am today because of all of you.

Sincerely,
Gabrielle Elise Jimenez

The daughter of a patient was sharing some stories of her mother as we sat at the bedside. I told her I loved hearing about my patients before they came under my care. I love to see photos of how they once looked, when they were healthy and strong. She told me that when it was my time to go, all of my patients, in their full glory would greet me. They will take my hand, they will hug me tightly and they will thank me for the love I gave them. And they will each sit me down and tell me about their lives before they met me and I will see them just as they were then.

I look very forward to that.

Printed in Great Britain
by Amazon